Esther

A Woman to be Reckoned With

"Simple Truths"
Esther: A Woman To Be Reckoned With

Linda Jones-White

ISBN- 13: 978-0-692-07694-1
ISBN: 1-69207-694-1

Unless noted otherwise, Scripture quotations are taken
from the King James Version (KJV) of the Holy Bible.

Published by Crawford Education Plus.

Cover design by LaVonne Booker.

Printed in the United States of America.

Esther

A Woman to be Reckoned With

Linda Jones-White

Crawford
EDUCATION PLUS

$\mathcal{W}$ith Much Thanks!

God, thanks so much for choosing me to be used as a vessel on Your behalf!

Kevin, thanks for always being loving and supportive for our entire 29 years of marriage!

Carolyn, you're a blessing as well as an encourager, and my biggest cheerleader. Thanks, Sis!

Pastors Ray and Tracey Barnard, my spiritual parents at Impacting Your World Christian Center Philadelphia, PA and Cherry Hill, NJ, thanks for all your diligence in your teachings!

Autumn Marie Cherry, much thanks to you for simply everything! God has crossed our paths for His glory! Words cannot express my gratitude for all you do!

$\mathscr{T}$able of Contents

Introduction

The Bible, the inspired Word of God, contains many nuggets or "simple truths" that can totally transform your life. One such truth can be found in the book of Esther.

Read the condensed story in this book of how Esther became queen, and note the parallels in your life!

As you continually draw closer to your King, you will experience more and more of His favor; and in His favor is life (Psalm 30:5)!

So, why Esther? And, what makes Esther a woman to be reckoned with?

Simply this: She obtained "favor" from the King.

To "favor" means to give special regard; to treat with goodwill; to show exceptional kindness or generosity.

Favor can lead to preferential treat-ment, as was the case with Esther.

Esther received royal favor above all the other virgins (Esther 2:17).

Favor may not always arrive in a material or worldly manner. God's favor may often come in the form of spiritual bless-ings, such as supernatural protection, or petitions being granted, even by ungodly civil authorities (Esther 7:3).

Favor can also cause policies, rules, and regulations to be changed or reversed to our advantage.

"If it please the king, and if I have favour in his sight, and the thing seem right before the king, and I be pleasing in his eyes, let it be written to reverse the letters devised by Haman the son of Hammedatha the Agagite, which he wrote to destroy the Jews which are in all the king's provinces" (Esther 8:5).

Read the following brief account of Esther's favor, and see how this simple truths can apply to your life today!

Chapter 1

Removal of Queen Vashti

During the time of Queen Esther, King Ahasuerus (Xerxes) reigned from India to Ethiopia in over 127 provinces. In these days, the king sat on his royal throne in the palace. It was simply beautiful!

During his third year as king, he threw a huge party for all of his staff, including the biggies. He showed them all the beautiful treasures and the rich and famous lifestyle he was living.

This celebration feast lasted seven whole days. Everything was overflowing including food and drinks. It was beautiful. There were precious pieces of tapestry made with the finest materials, marble pillows, couches of gold and silver, and all rested on the best pavements. It was a sight to behold.

The king's display included the best quality of precious gemstones too. During this time the drinks continued to be served in the finest goblets, including only the best royal wine.

At the same time of the king's celebration, Queen Vashti was having a celebration for all the women located in another room in the palace. After an entire week of celebrating and when the king's heart was very "happy" with wine, he asked one of his court to bring Queen Vashti to him with her royal crown on her head, so he could show her off to all his guests. Upon the queen receiving the message on the behalf of the king, the queen sent a return message to the king that she refused to come to him. This was unheard of! When the king received the return message, he was furious. He did not know what to do, so he started talking to several of the persons at the party asking, "What should I do?"

They all concurred that this could not be allowed and had to be stopped immediately. To ensure that this behavior, by women, would never happen again, it was suggested that she be made

an al of. A suggestion was made to the
king to divorce her right away and separate
from her that same day. So that's what the king
did. And Queen Vashti was removed from her
position and from the palace that same day.

Chapter 2

Esther Chosen as Queen

Now all the responsibility to find a new queen would be on Hegai, who was in charge of the entire process from beginning to end. This process would take one full year.

Now there was a certain Jew named Mordecai who had a niece whose mother and father had died; he raised her as his daughter. Her name was Esther. She was lovely. Esther, one of the women chosen, was taken to the king's palace and given to Hegai. Mordecai instructed Esther to follow all Hegai's instructions and to follow them exactly as they were given. Mordecai reiterated again and again to Esther to remember to do everything told so she could be pleasing to the king.

Esther pleased Hegai and received favor from him. He quickly gave her all the essentials needed right from the start and placed her with the first group that would see the king. That included the best living accommodations.

Mordecai reiterated again and Mordecai instructed her never to reveal her nationality for any reason to anyone.

Mordecai was an attendant at the king's gate, so daily he would watch and see Esther and get updates on how she was doing. Of course, no one ever knew their real relationship.

All the women had to be just right before they would meet with the king. So the women continued their extensive 12-month process. During this process they had beauty treatments which consisted of six months of oil and myrrh, and six months with sweet spices and per-fumes. All of this was the ongoing purify-ing for the women. By the end of this whole regiment the women would b full prepared for their visit with the king in his palace. They would each go in during evening and return the next morning. After being with the king, each candidate would not return to the king unless he requested to see her again.

When Esther's turn came to go to the king, she immediately won favor in his sight. Esther received favor in so many ways. Instead of a 12-month process for the king, she went only 10 months. She also received favor when the king set the crown on her head as his new choice for new queen. The king had a great feast and all the maidens and Mordecai sat at the front gate to watch.

Plot to Kill King Ashasuerus

During these days while Mordecai was at the gate, he heard two of the king's officers plotting to kill the king. He got a message to Queen Esther and told her to warn the king about the plot to kill him. It was investigated and found to be true. The officers were hung in the gallows. It was written in the book of chronicles, right in front of the king.

Chapter 3

Haman's Plot Against
the Jews

In the meantime, King Ahasuerus promoted Haman. Haman's seat was above all the other princes and all of the other servants at the gate. They all bowed down to Haman, except Mordecai. The king's servants asked Mordecai again why he would not bow down. They continued to ask, but Mordecai did not respond. He continued to pay them no attention and just kept doing what he was supposed to be doing. So Haman, once finding out by his officers they shared the nationality of Mordecai, which is Jewish, became very angry and decided to get even for Mordecai not bowing down to him. Haman decided to destroy all the Jews because of the actions of Mordecai.

Haman told King Ahasuerus that certain people had different laws than him, and that they weren't keeping the king's laws. It is not in his best intrest to allow this to continue. He asked for the king's permission to decree that all the Jews be destroyed. The king took his signet ring, which was used to sign and seal letters, giving the authority to Haman. And Haman wrote the letters and called all the necessary staff to come and distribute the letters all over the king's provinces to destroy and do away with all Jews. This included both young and old, as well as women and children. This was published and a decree given to all people to read.

Chapter 4

Mordecai Asks Esther
for Help

When Mordecai heard of what was being planned, he was furious. He tore off his regular uniform that he wore at the gate in front of the king's palace and put on a sack cloth with dirty ashes and went to the city and cried out loudly. He positioned himself right in front of the king's gate. Now no one would ever enter the king's gate dressed like that. Once the letter was received at all the provinces, the people (Jews) were very sad, crying, fasting and many wore sack cloths and ashes.

When Esther's maids told her they saw Mordecai and what he was wearing at the gate, she was so upset. She sent new garments by her staff down to him, but he refused to take them.

Esther called one of the king's attendants, which the king had given to her, whose name was Hathach. Esther asked Hathach to go to Mordecai and find out what was wrong. Mordecai shared everything with him concerning the decree that Haman had distributed to destroy all Jews. He told him to tell Esther she must go to the king and plead on their behalf. Hathach returned to the queen, giving her all the information from Mordecai.

Queen Esther listened and sent a message back to Mordecai saying, "I cannot go in to see the king without being personally summoned by Him. I could be put to death. He has not called for me in thirty days."

Again Hathach returned from Mordecai with this message: "Don't think so high of yourself that you are not a part of this decree also. Let me remind you that you to are still a Jew. You can't keep silent at this time. Relief and deliverance shall arise from elsewhere, but you and your father's house will perish. Who knows that you were not placed here for such a time as this!"

Esther sent Hathach back to Mordecai with this reply: "Gather all the Jews together and fast on my behalf for the next three days. Do not eat or drink during that time. My staff and I will also do the same and then I will go to the king, and if I perish I will perish."

So Mordecai went and did all he was instructed to do.

Chapter 5

Esther's Intervention

On the third day of the fast, Esther put on her special royal attire and stood in the royal court of the king's palace. The king was delighted when he saw Queen Esther, who obtained favor. He held out his scepter to her hand, motioning her to come to him.

The king asked his queen what she would like today... "Whatever it is, it shall be done!" the king said, "Even if it's half of my kingdom, its yours!"

She said, "I'd like Haman to come and have dinner with us, and I will prepare it for us."

He said, "It's done!"

So the king and Haman came to the dinner that Esther prepared. During dinner the king asked again to his queen, "What is your request?"

Esther said, "King, my request is: If it's okay with you, let Haman come to dinner tomorrow and have dinner with us again, and I will prepare the food."

And the king agreed. Haman went away happy and excited. But little did he know when he saw Mordecai at the gate, all the anger came up against him again.

Haman was basically bragging to people about all he and his family had, including his promotion which elevated him above all the other princes and servants of the king. Haman also shared that he had dinner that day with the king and queen and was going to return and have dinner again tomorrow. He was so excited and pleased thinking he was above and better then all everyone else.

Haman has Gallows Made

Haman also discussed with his wife Zeresh, as well as his friends, the situation with Mordecai. They agreed that Haman should build a gallows and give specifics in the morning to the king. He wanted to suggest that Haman be hung on it. He liked the idea and said the gallows would be built.

Chapter 6

Mordecai Honored

That night the king was very restless when he went to bed. He normally had no problem sleeping, but this night he did. He ordered a book to be brought to him and read. While being read to, he learned where Mordecai had told of the two who were plotting to kill him. The king asked what honor was given to Mordecai for sharing this information and keeping his life safe. "Nothing," was the reply from his servant. The king asked who was in the court now. Haman had just entered into the court at the exact time the servant was asked who was in the court. The king's servant answered, "Haman is there."

So Haman came into the king's presence.

The king asked Haman, "What should I do for the person who did not receive honor from a good deed done on my behalf?"

Haman, of course, thought he was talking about him, and was so happy!

"Well," he said, "Let him receive royal clothes and a horse that you have ridden on. Also, let a royal crown be placed upon his head. Let him ride on the open square amongst the entire city, being shown to all. This is what I suggest should be done."

And the king agreed.

So Haman hurried and took the clothes and horse and began proclaiming before him, this shall be done to the man who the king delights to honor.

Then the king requested to take Mordecai off the gate. Haman left sad and upset, with his head down. Haman went and talked with his wife and friends telling them how everything had changed. So they told him to go back and repent and ask for forgiveness to save his life.

While they were still talking the king's attendant came and said that the king asked for him to come before his presence. And quickly Haman went back with him for the dinner with the king and queen which she had prepared.

Chapter 7

Downfall of Haman

So the king, Haman and the queen all dined together for the second day. The king asked for the second day and the second time, "What is your request? And I will grant it!"

And again he said, "If it's half of my kingdom, it's yours."

The queen said, "If it pleases you, let my life be given and the lives of my people be spared."

The king asked the queen, "Who dares to do this?"

"A very evil person—Haman," she said.

Now Haman was very afraid, as he sat in the presence of both the king and queen. The king got up from his chair very angry. He left and went into his garden to calm down and think clearly before making a decision. Haman jumped up and went to the queen and made a plea for his life. On the return of the king, Haman was on the couch with the queen. This more infuriated the king. He immediately asked his queen if he had forced himself on her. No, she answered.

The king said, "Hang him!"

The servant covered Haman's face and hung him on the same gallows he had made for Mordecai. Once done, the king was satisfied.

Chapter 8

Decree Revoked

On this day the king gave his queen the house of Haman. Mordecai, on the same day, went to the king and told him the relationship between Queen Esther and him. After the talk with the king, the king took off his ring and gave it to Mordecai. Esther placed Mordecai over the house of Haman.

Notice how God turned the tables around.

Esther spoke to the king and fell at his feet and asked him to stop the plot to kill all the Jews. She told him about the horrible scheme set up by Haman to kill all the Jews. She asked, if it pleased him, if he would rescind the previous letter sent to all the provinces. He agreed and letters were sent out with the king's signet stamp to all the provinces to rescind the original decree to kill of the Jews. Need-less to say, the Jews were very happy after finding out that their lives were being saved.

Happiness and excitement spread fast to all!

Shortly thereafter a feast and holiday celebration took place, all the Jews knew that favor was granted and had fallen on them.

Chapter 9

Victory of the Jews

The battle came to those against the Jews on the same day that the Jews were to be executed and it turned around for the good. The tables turned. That's how God can and will change any and all situations quickly! The Jews gathered together and took their rightful place again and began anew.

Mordecai was great in the king's palace and people knew him throughout. He became more and more powerful, so much so that those who hated against him were destroyed.

There were ten sons of Haman's left behind who hated the Jews.

The king asked the queen, "What should we do with them?"

The queen said, "If it's okay with you, I would like the dead bodies of Haman's sons to be hanged on gallows."

The king said, "It is so granted."

Mordecai recorded all the activities of all the Jews all over. Then he forwarded letters to the Jews in all of the king's provinces. These two days were made annual days of rest, gratitude, gifts to the poor, and celebration for the Jews to remem-ber always. The Jews ordained that these two days every year must be never for-gotten and passed down to all their chil-dren and children's children, for all gen-erations to come.

The queen gave full power to the second letter written in words of peace and truth. And all was confirmed, written, and kept in the book.

Chapter 10

Greatness of Mordecai

The king decreed taxes must be paid on the land and sea. Now Mordecai, a Jew, was held in high esteem and was second in command next to the king.

Mordecai was great among his people. He was a favorite with them all. He always made sure the best welfare was made on behalf of his people and spoke peace to his entire nationality.

$\mathscr{A}$ SIMPLE TRUTH

What makes Esther a woman to be reckoned with?
Simply this: Esther is a woman to be reckoned with because of her faithfulness, humility, and knowledge of the power of prayer and fasting in God! That is how Esther obtained "favor" from the King.
Let God use you to find your "SIMPLE TRUTHS" and let your mind be transformed through the renewing process.

Romans 12:2

"And be ye not conformed to this world: but be ye transformed by the renewing of your mind, that you may prove what is that good, and acceptable, and perfect will of God."
King James Version (KJV)

$\mathcal{A}$bout the Author

Linda Jones-White: Who is she? A Woman of God, chosen by God, for such a time as this! My favorite scripture sums it up: For God knows the thoughts and plans he has for me (Jeremiah 29:11).

As I long to continue to stay in God's will for my life, He has truly ordered my steps! He allows me to blossom in Him through more and more gifts: As an entrepreneur of two businesses, Sisters N Crafts LLC, a Personalized Gift Basket Service, and a Mary Kay Consultant, as well as Author, Life Coach and Mentor. God is so good to me!

Compassionate Women of Destiny, International (CWODI) is a women's monthly Bible study fellowship birthed by God. CWODI reaches numerous women of all backgrounds, ages, races, and denominations. One of the key mandates is to be able to share with women who have been hurt in the traditional church setting and have no desire to return. I am able to teach "simple truths," which mean practical biblical teachings through God's Word to develop and grow women. My vision for CWODI is to reach, teach and touch women of all ages, backgrounds and lifestyles, leading them by example that being saved and satisfied in Him really works!

My goal in life is to excel in the destiny God has for me. I have been married twenty nine years to the first and only love of my life, Kevin L. White. Kevin continues to allow me to spread my wings to do what God calls me to do. I am also truly blessed to have several spiritual daughters, an encouraging family, and numerous loving, caring and sharing support systems.

"Simple Truths" is shared with those of you who really care to grow spiritually in God's will! Enjoy the experience!

Other books available by the author, Linda Jones-White

Fruit of the Spirit Journal

Birthing by God's Supernatural Provision

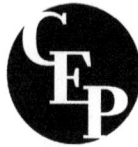

Crawford
EDUCATION PLUS

Books forthcoming
by the author

Blessings or Curses: You Choose!

Sharing Praise Thru Psalms

Conversations with God Daily

Seasons of Preparation

Blessings, Favor & Increase Journal

Fruit of the Spirit Study Guide

A Virtuous Woman

www.ingramcontent.com/pod-product-compliance
Lightning Source LLC
Chambersburg PA
CBHW070803300326
41914CB00052B/643